HOW I CONQUERED MY HEADACHES

I. INTRODUCTION

A. WHAT IS CLUSTER HEADACHE SYNDROME?

This book is an accounting of my living with **"The Cluster Headache Syndrome",** and the battle my wife and I waged to overcome this severe handicap. I am not a doctor, and therefore not able to make medical recommendations, write prescriptions, or otherwise assist people with the same or like problems. I make no claims to anyone that I have conducted exhaustive scientific research on this subject. My sole purpose in writing this book is that it is possible I may be able to benefit some unfortunate soul who suffers from cluster or non-cluster headaches by relating to my extensive experience and analysis.

If you are a cluster headache sufferer you are quite aware of the mighty few written references available that have proved effective. I simply am trying to let other people in the same situation as I was in, understand that there are preventive techniques that they can employ to prevent the headaches. There are few, if any, authoritative and

1

helpful discussions of the people who have been afflicted. Most of the "cures" have come from people who have never had a cluster headache. By way of explanation, the "Cluster Headache Syndrome" is limited to one person of every 221,000 population or roughly four people in a million.

This book is written in three sections; (1) An Introduction, (2) The attempts my wife and I made to get at the root cause of the disease. Also, what didn't work, and (3) How I Finally Solved the Problem Through Prevention. My wife called these food and beverage diets, "triggers" in the case. "Avoid the "triggers", as there is nothing anyone can do to stop the headaches once they have started", was her favorite saying. HOW PROPHETIC SHE WAS!!!

These headaches are so complex and complicated that you cannot prevent them with a few words of advice. Please read to the end of this book to fully understand this almost indecipherable dilemma.

The pain is the most severe known to man. It is recognized that 2/3 of all people who have experienced this complex syndrome have committed suicide. That would be the easy way out. I had a friend who just couldn't live with the pain anymore, got awfully drunk and attempted to end his life. He was unsuccessful, living with a bullet lodged in his skull until he died at a ripe old age. There are few old headache sufferers. This is unfortunate since it takes a lifetime of analysis to get to the bottom of the cause of the disease.

This is what a member of the Worldwide Support Group wrote about his affliction: *"I've just gotten over an attack. I've been going 5 weeks now non-stop. 4-6 attacks per day. No sleep. No relief. I'm exhausted. I keep telling myself this hell is going to end soon, but I'm beginning to think that it's not. I can't think. I can't eat. I can't leave my house. When I'm not in pain, I'm in dread of it coming back. The attacks are increasing in intensity everyday and I sometimes think that I will go mad. I try everything to ease them a little and nothing seems to be working. I really don't know how much more I can take.*

I keep telling myself that I am strong enough to deal with it. I've been doing it for a long time now. But then the next one hits, and I become a whimpering little baby with no strength what so ever. My only saving grace is being able to write this down and know that you will understand like no one else can. I'll close my eyes now and hope that maybe I will sleep a little before the next one hits. Thanks for being here."

- *Marcus*

It started about 2 A.M. I was awakened from my sleep with this burning sensation in my ear and back of my neck. I tried to shift positions and return to my peaceful sleep, but it wasn't happening. Something in my mind told me immediately that I was dealing with the same crap I did a couple of years ago, and even though I tried to convince myself that it wasn't the same, I KNEW it was.

My right eye felt like it took a couple punches, and my right nostril was starting to leak. I got out of bed, and went downstairs, all the while, this pressure in the right side of my brain kept building and building. My right eyelid was beginning to swell shut. I was squinting and it was tearing. I kept looking at the tears coming out of my eyes, convinced there was blood pouring out. I dropped to the floor and pressed my hands so hard against my temples that I thought I was going to crush my skull, it wasn't helping. I got up and well, I went insane. It's the only thing I think I can describe it...stark raving lunatic insane!

Cluster Headaches take over your life completely. Don't expect anyone to be sympathetic or empathetic to your plight. It is not possible for anyone to understand the level of pain anymore than it is possible for a normal person to appreciate back pain, or a toothache because they have not experienced it. An old Indian proverb states the case well, "Do not judge a man until you have walked a mile in his sandals". Doctors will almost always quiz you on the intensity of the pain on a scale of 1 to 10; ten being the most severe. Cluster and migraine headaches are almost always in the 8 to 10 bracket, which means unbearable.

It is not inherited and is not contagious. (You can't get it from anyone else). It simply is a disease that you have or you don't. You have to be lucky to be one of four in a million to have it when you are born. It is designated non-fatal, but I wondered many times if the constant expanding of the blood vessels might cause them to burst.

Being a staunch Christian, and even after losing about a third of my life to this disease, I never contemplated taking my life, because God knows I have this affliction, and He never gives people heavier crosses than they can bear. As hard as it is to understand, the Good Lord always has a reason. Every person in the world has some health problem, some worse than others. No one is perfect. But life is entirely too precious to waste with a bullet. Think of all the wonderful blessings we enjoy when we are healthy.

II.   MY LIFE LONG STRUGGLE

A. EARLY BEGINNING

My earliest recollection of my personal affliction began at approximately age five. (When most people can first start to remember incidences). Standing at the foot of my bed while my mother straightened it, I suddenly felt a very stinging, penetrating pain over my left eye. My mother asked, "What's wrong?" I answered, "I've got a headache and fainted!" When I awoke, I found my mother had laid me on the newly made bed, and was putting washcloths on my forehead, which had been soaked with cold well water. We had no refrigerator. She seemed greatly relieved when I opened my eyes. As has happened for the next seventy-five years, she said I was as white as a ghost and she was deathly afraid I wouldn't wake up.

My mother treated all our illnesses with two standard medications; aspirin and physics. Whether you needed bowel movement insurance was inconsequential; she felt it would help whatever ailed you. (Ironically, there have been numerous articles actually recommending this as a treatment to relieve cluster headaches)

Eventually, it became apparent that this affliction was interfering with my job performance. I never confided about this with anyone but my wife. I tried to hide it because it was so misunderstood even by me. The local eye, ear, and nose specialists had nothing to offer, so I sought advanced medical advice at Madison, WI General Hospital operated by the University of Wisconsin. Upon arrival I went through the usual routine of analysis of my "condition" by an admitting doctor. It didn't take long for her to come to the conclusion that I did not have a flawed sinus condition. She was emphatic about it.

" Discontinue all treatments you are taking for sinuses," she said. "They have already done enough damage to the bones in your nose passages. I am sending you to our senior neurologist." And off I went.

Another more complete battery of tests was ordered including brain wave, to determine if any tumors were present. In my interview with the neurologist the next day, he said, "The good news is, you don't have any tumors. The bad news is you have what we call "Cluster Headaches" and there is no known treatment. But we do know this. Only men with Type A personality are afflicted. These are people like you who put extra pressure on themselves for achievement and accomplishment. They haven't learned how to relax and have fun. Their work is the center of their lives; that's all they do and care about" He could have said stress and it would have summed up everything he told me. I had recently taken up golf, and sought to relieve my stress at every opportunity. It resolved nothing. He had the right name for the problem, but the wrong way to cure it.

B.   AT LAST AN UNDERSTANDING OF THE PROBLEM

This account is not intended to malign the medical profession; only to point out how little is known about this disease. It is not surprising that there was no knowledge of this syndrome in the 1930's, as it took until the year 2001, that a neurologist outlined a definitive cause for the headaches in a national press conference. He had the brilliant idea to hospitalize patients so they could inform him immediately when an episode began. He piped their blood through a high-powered microscope in order to get a first hand observation of what was happening to them. He made the history-making discovery that their normally round blood cells were changing shape. They became trapezoids, rectangles and all other odd shapes. Unable to get through the small capillaries leading to the brain, (the body's smallest blood vessels), forced them to expand which caused the severe pain that accompanied this event. As the heart continued to put pressure on the system to force blood through these vessels, they were expanding and the pain increased.

When queried by reporters, he cautioned that a cure was a long ways off. He continued to comment, "At this time, the medical profession has no idea how blood enters the circulatory system. If it is manufactured in the bone marrow as is widely acclaimed, how does it get out of the bone, where it is completely enclosed? After we learn all that, then we need to get to the source of the blood with a medication that will prevent cell shape change. This could take many years, and I would not wish to make a forecast on how long!" He might have added, that with a total of only a few hundred over a thousand cluster headache sufferers in the United States, which funds most of the world's research, the market is entirely too small for any pharmaceutical company to do any amount of exhaustive research on this subject. With millions of heart and cancer patients, the chances of a company taking up this cause are mighty slim indeed.

C. DOCTORS ETHICS WHEN THERE IS NO HOPE

There will always be diseases for which there is no cure. But if I were a doctor, the very last thing I would wish to tell a suffering patient is that there is nothing we can do for you. You would want to give them hope. But the doctor has to be careful not to cross the line of prudence, when in his experience with other patients with the same problems proves his treatments are fruitless. If told there is nothing that the doctor can do, most patients would seek other opinions and look for other options or resign themselves to their fate, rather than keep visiting the same doctor for years without results.

Some patients rely solely on their family doctor's opinion, while others feel they are in charge of their own health and well being. I continued to seek advice at the foremost clinics in the Midwest. Some said they did not attempt to treat cluster headaches. Others gave me many different drugs to try. Some were intended for other diseases and made the headaches drastically worse. I tried over fifty different drugs. As I learned more about steroids, I was more determined not to take them. The side effects were awful and the long-term consequences were not appealing.

1. TRIGGERS ARE KEY

This became a lightning rod for my wife, Carole, as she concluded and probably rightly so, that any chance of a "cure" was more remote than ever. She insisted that the need to find the "triggers" was more imperative than before. We both felt that somehow, what I ate and drank had a direct bearing on this.

This becomes a mind-boggling exercise, as we hardly ever, if at all, sustain ourselves with only one substance. You could make bread with only flour and water, but it would not be a rounded out diet. And pretty tiresome. Practically everything you eat has more than one element, with the exception of bananas, eggs, apples, nuts, and a few other foods. But no one food can supply all the vitamins and energy our bodies require. It takes a well-rounded list of foods to supply ample nutrition.

The headaches continued as I grew up. One of the more unexplainable facets about them is that if I was awakened at 2:10 A.M., awaking me from a sound sleep without warning, they continued that identical pattern regardless of when I went to sleep. I guarantee you could set watch by it. This is one of the methods that is used to separate cluster headaches from other more common types. Another distinguishing characteristic of this syndrome is that the pain is so concentrated in one spot. In my case, it was just above my left eye. The pain never ceases completely; if touched it is tender, sore, and very painful.

At first, there were intermittent periods when they were in submission. Sometimes a year or two went by before I experienced an episode of constant, pounding, throbbing, pains, which always came on very suddenly and did not respond to any painkillers. Of course, during this remission period I could lead a normal life, but continued to amass a collection of every article that appeared in newspapers, magazines, television and radio that pertained to "miraculous cures" regardless of how bizarre they appeared. As I got older, there wasn't any period of remission. They were almost constant and I had become immune to most painkillers.

B. THE "EXPERTS" ON CLUSTER HEADACHES

It seems that everyone except the person who suffers the headaches has a "cure" that's as simple as ABC. I had certain teeth extracted, had my head covered with special materials, got rid of feather pillows and replaced them with foam rubber. Mostly their claims were centered on reducing or eliminating the pain through the use of tons of different types of salves, lidocaine drops, hot baths, elevating the head of the bed, heat and ultraviolet lamps, exercise, sleeping in the cold, and many other pipe dreams all of which I tried to no avail.

Somewhere in my long history of collecting articles about headache relief, I had read that oxygen was THE thing. The doctor gave me a prescription for a tank and breathing device, which I used frequently. All hoaxes. None of them recommended preventive measures. Naturally all victims are desperate and will try anything, as there was no known medication for it.

C.   WE TRIED EVERYTHING

Someone wrote a book on the hazards of using processed white sugars. My wife wanted me to give it a try. As desperate as I was, I would give anything if the motivation were strong enough. Having a sweet tooth, it was like giving up my right arm to give up all use of sugar. My wife had an unbelievably hard time cooking and baking for seven people as it was, without eliminating sugar for my consumption. Year-around fasting from the diet I was raised on. But I did it for four years. I bought ice cream made with honey, as that was not a processed sugar. And it worked for those years, but eventually, it too failed. But I am sure now it is one of many substances that are "triggers". However, to give credit where credit is due, it was the longest period in my life without a headache. I am not sure if it was the sugar or the lack of processing.

In more recent recommendations, it is claimed that processing meats, sausages, wieners, bratwurst, lunch meats, ham, cheeses, pickles, onions, olives, certain types of beans, raisins, avocados, canned soups, and red wine are high in teramines, which by themselves are sufficient to cause the "triggers" to activate. The Cleveland Headache Clinic warns against eating the following types of cheese: Blue cheese, Brie, Cheddar, Stilton, Feta, Gorgonzola, Mozzarella, Muenster, Parmesan, Swiss, and Processed cheese.

Certain food additives, including nitrates are also common headaches triggers. I have never noticed any effect from eating canned or frozen fruits and vegetables. Some people have identified nuts, cheese, and wine, as the "three amigos" that cause all the trouble. Later on, MSG was branded as a headache provoker along with preservatives. Of course, alcohol or liquor is a no-no as well as smoking. Second hand smoke being as bad as the smoking itself

D. OXYGEN

The use of oxygen has long been recommended. I had abbreviated success with it. Deep breathing exercises are just as effective. It takes a long period of time to achieve a measure of success, as longer than a half hour of deep breathing can be very difficult.

E. IMITREX

For a period it appeared as if Imitrex was the wonder drug that would magically take care of them, but alas, it only postponed the headaches a few hours. Even ignoring the dosage of certain over-the-counter medications, for if you died, that was OK, because the headaches were unbearable anyway. Only about five per cent of doctors would tackle the problem. If they did, they had put together some kind of weird combinations of drugs of which the security of the patient was in doubt. Or else they simply said it was a sinus problem. In my case, one doctor cracked the bones on the inside of my nose to open the passages. Almost as bad as the headache. Chiropractors tried to straighten out the neck by putting my head on a box and kneeling on my neck. When the bones started to sound like they were cracking, I ran for the door. Of course, I had been to Madison University Hospital at which it was determined I had no sinus problem. I fell back on over-the-counter medications as nobody had an answer or was able to help. Even now, it is safe to say that ninety-five percent of doctors cannot identify "The Cluster Headache Syndrome".

E. PAINKILLERS

The neurologist I was seeing recommended I use one Tylenol 3 every four hours. When I went to see a $500/hour specialist, he recommended Two Tylenol 3's every one-half hour until the headache subsided. One every four hours would only guarantee that the headache would remain. That info was really worth $500.00 as it was the only painkiller that accomplished anything, even though I was at times taking the equivalent of 36 regular Tylenols every three hours.

When Prednisone became available, my doctor prescribed 60 mg./day for a week, then 50 per day for a week, and so on until it got down to 2 ½ mg./day for the last two weeks. For a total of 1565 mg. per year. For those who have never used prednisone, it is a steroid which has a myriad of side effects, principal of which is incessant hunger, puffing of the face, losing your balance, acting as if you might be under the influence, extreme sleeplessness, great anxiety, like the feeling of walking about three feet off the ground, leg and finger cramps so severe you have to pry your fingers one by one off the steering wheel, bleeding profusely from the slightest scratch, and just feeling listless like a continual flu. Sometimes it worked and broke the cycle of the headache episode. It was most effective at the higher dosage, and many times the headaches returned when the dosage got below 40 mg./day.

It should be mentioned here that there is more to this disease than an uncontrollable headache. Sometimes it is completely incapacitating leaving you unable to even move your arms. Now that we know the cause, it is not at all surprising this happens when the blood flow is so restricted.

II. SOLVING THE PROBLEM THROUGH PREVENTION

A. YOU MUST HAVE THE CONVICTION THAT YOU ARE IN CHARGE OF YOUR OWN HEALTH.

That's absolutely essential. In this critical time of your life, you cannot afford to let a doctor practice on your misfortune. For him, it's like playing roulette. If he wins, he will be recognized as a great physician in the whole United States medical community. If he loses, nothing happens. You have paid him for being a practicing physician. You are the loser, for you have lost valuable time. TIME is the greatest thing you have in your life. When it is gone, it is gone forever and can never be retrieved. Regardless of how many drugs are prescribed, do not be content, for this is a disease that does not respond to pills.

> YOU MUST PREVENT THE HEADACHES WITH ALL THE SPIRIT AND WILL POWER YOU CAN MUSTER. PAINKILLERS ARE NOT THE ANSWER. THE RESPONSIBILITY FOR YOUR HEALTH LIES WITH YOU.

In the short time you spend with the doctor or neurologist you see, he cannot determine what's best for you unless it's some run-of-the-mill disease like the flu. Cluster Headaches are a highly specialized type of disease. It demands every bit of your talent and ingenuity. Analyze, analyze, and analyze some more. This book should help you, as it gives you the benefit of 75 years of analysis, with little or no help from doctors. Most of them discouraged checking diets. They would rather treat the symptoms and forget preventive medicine. Thought they could conquer the pain with pills.

The beauty of this analysis is that you don't have to take anything. NO PILLS. It is all about taking away some things you may like, use all the will power you can muster, and learn to manage your life.

B. THE BREAKTHROUGH

THE BASIS OF ALL RESEARCH IS TO
"ELIMINATE THE VARIABLES"

IN ORDER TO ELIMINATE THE VARIABLES, MEANS THAT YOU MUST EAT OR DRINK ONLY ONE SUBSTANCE AT A TIME. IT WILL NOT WORK TO TAKE AWAY ONE SUBSTANCE AT A TIME. YOU MUST ADD ONE SUBSTANCE AT A TIME AFTER YOU HAVE ASCERTAINED THAT WHAT YOU ARE EATING OR DRINKING IS SAFE.

It all happened by accident. I had purchased a gallon of cranraspberry juice. One day I had my own home made bread toasted and a poached egg, my last resort diet. I had headaches almost every day for three years. Actually I did this diet numerous times for a week or more at a time, to make sure I wasn't getting anything that would further promote the headaches. This would abate the severity of the pain somewhat. This generally worked as I used skim milk for a beverage, shunning coffee or sodas. I also felt safe in drinking the cranraspberry juice since the ingredients indicated the juice contained only water, cranberry, and raspberry. Since I had run out of milk, I poured a glass of the cranraspberry, which I thoroughly enjoyed. Within fifteen minutes, I had a knockdown cluster headache, Unbelievably severe. I took two Tylenol 3's(1500 mg each acetaminophen with codeine) immediately, and again in a half hour I repeated the dosage. And another half hour after that, and again in another half hour. That's the equivalent of 24 Tylenols in two hours, and it made no impact on my headache." That's too much," I said to myself, and didn't take anymore even though my head was pounding. Sometimes oxygen has helped, so I sat out in the screen porch for the rest of the night wrapped in a comforter, as the temperature hovered near 40. I practiced deep breathing and put an ice pack on my head. It may be my imagination that this helps, but when you are in a desperate situation, you will try anything to relieve the blinding, agonizing pain.

The next day I was unable to function so I had plenty of time to contemplate what had gone wrong. I reviewed the list of ingredients. Nothing different. Really had me stumped. I continued with the toasted home made bread and egg diet with an occasional banana. Two weeks later, out with company we stopped for an ice cream sundae. Confident that vanilla ice cream posed no problem, I also had a pineapple topping. I thought,

" Natural fruit can't be harmful." After eating that, and we had not yet left the ice cream parlor, I again was jolted with a terrible headache. I had to have someone take me back to my motel.

I repeated the Tylenol dosage as before and had lots of time to peruse the situation. What could possibly have happened? How were the two incidents connected? What was the trigger in these cases? Later, I had a bottle of cola, and again the same reaction! Another severe headache. None of these things were on my avoidance list. The cola can had the usual ingredients. Nothing prohibitive. So what caused the headache? Stumped again!!

But after a lifetime of analysis, I was sure there was a connection between the three incidents, as my toast and milk diet was too exclusive to allow for a headache. I was wishing Carole were there to help me. Here were three innocuous substances, which by themselves would never be under suspicion of causing the dreaded symptoms. But each one did. Wracking my brain for a solution, to no avail I again reviewed the labels. I was left to my own ingenuity to decipher what had gone wrong. I looked at every item individually and thought long and hard. Unfortunately, I was living alone in a rented house and couldn't bounce ideas off anyone. Nobody to turn to for conversation, consultation, or help dig into the dilemma. There was no easy solution, as cluster headache syndrome is as complex as Winston Churchill said about the Soviet Union. A riddle within an enigma wrapped up in a puzzle. Many smarter and better-educated people than me had analyzed this to death and came up empty. By and large, all the research was directed toward ridding the patient of the headache. They were looking for drugs to stymie pain messages from getting through to the brain. Both my wife and I stubbornly held to the theory that as long as no one else had solved the mystery with his or her approaches, it had to lay in a less complicated answer. Namely, food and beverage intake.

Then it hit me like a ton of brick. Suddenly I realized that as I stared at the cranraspberry juice, it was **TOO RED.** I had seen cranberries harvested. They are orange, pink, white, yellow, but **not** a beautiful red color. Even raspberries are not all red. So, no matter how much raspberry juice they added, they could not make the whole gallon a beautiful red. They added food coloring!!!! Then I thought about the fact that when the girl making my ice cream sundae was pumping out the pineapple topping, it was just **TOO GOLDEN.** I had seen pineapples harvested in Hawaii. They are not all golden in color. Again I deciphered that food coloring had been added. The cola was a **light brown.** Not water colored which is basically what cola is. The next week in a theater, Coca-Cola had an ad on the screen, which indicated they were the sole suppliers of cola to this chain and that all their products had added color.

I immediately took inventory of everything I was eating and drinking and found mighty few items that were not colored. I continued to narrow my diet, eliminating every suspicious item. Such as mustard, catch-up, box cakes, pie fillings, puddings, Jell-O, cheddar cheese, (which has only one ounce per thousand pounds of milk), but is sufficient to cause a problem for me, butter, and on and on. Even meat is injected with a red dye. **Avoiding these has relieved me of all headaches since.**

Unfortunately, when my wife and I were checking ingredients for everything I ate, we didn't know that companies are exempt from listing ingredients that comprise less than 2% of the total substance. So dyes are seldom, if ever, listed.

C. FOOD AND BEVERAGE INGREDIENTS

IN ORDER TO DETERMINE WHICH FOODS WOULD BE SAFE TO EAT OR DRINK, I SENT A LETTER TO MOST OF THE MAJOR COMPANIES, WITH THE FOLLOWING INQUIRY:

Dear Sirs: RE: ALLERGIES

Please do not misconstrue my intent in requesting information. I am extremely allergic to many types of food flavors, coloring, flavoring enhancers, etc. I merely wish to avoid those that affect me. Since the FDA exempts an ingredient from being labeled when it comprises less than 2% of the total product, I have little or no opportunity in purchasing food items to determine if these additives are present. **The information I am seeking is a list of beverages or food that you market or produce, that do not contain MSG, preservatives, flavor enhancers, soy bean hydrogenated oil, sugar substitutes such as aspartame and any food coloring agents or dyes. Even though dyes are** used in minimal amounts, they apparently are the worst offenders in my case. I thought this list would be considerably shorter than one that did contain these substances. I am particularly interested in whether you use **MSG or food coloring in your meat products.** A victim of food poisoning, which damaged my stomach severely, while serving in the Armed Forces during World War II, has magnified my susceptibility to these types of products in recent years. Thanking you in advance for your cooperation.

Sincerely,

GENERAL Mill's Consumer Service Representative maintains that all their products list the three standard food colorings: Blue 1, Yellow 5 and Red 40 as well as soybean derivatives and preservatives, and aspartame.

EDY'S ICE CREAM: Failed to comment on the questions and sent a form indicating the size container in which each of their products is sold

CAMPBELL SOUP COMPANY'S representative replied, "Since product ingredients change frequently, we are unable to maintain current lists of products which do not contain certain ingredients. Please refer to the ingredient statement on each package for the most up to date information.

(Author's Comment: Our litigious society has led these companies to prefer not to answer any questions from consumers, regardless of the intent of the question).

C. NON-FOOD OR BEVERAGE PRODUCTS

1.   One product that always created a problem for me, was the type of hair spray or material used in giving permanent waves. My wife thought at times I was allergic to her, but it was only the hair spray.

CAUTION: You are bound to have periods when you can not figure out what gave you a headache. You will usually find that it was some little thing that you thought would have no effect on you. Something as insignificant as an 1/8th of a teaspoon of a condiment such as allspice in pumpkin pie, a axed cake, or a small bite of cheddar cheese. When it comes to food coloring, <u>none</u> is the only way to go. Not even a sip of soda. Be firm!! Let your friends know you can not tolerate <u>any</u> food coloring or seasoning. Use salt and pepper.

SO WHERE DOES THAT LEAVE US?

<u>**THE FOLLOWING PARAGRAPH IS THE MOST IMPORTANT INFORMATION YOU WILL EVER RECEIVE FROM ANY DOCTOR OR ANYBODY ELSE CONCERNING CLUSTER/MIGRAINE HEADACHES AS AFFECTED BY ALLERGIES:**</u>

All this information is what you need to prevent your headaches. Firstly, I think cluster headache, migraine headache, although having a slightly different imprint of each person who unfortunately suffers from them, can be looked at as basically the same, and will respond to the same preventative treatment. These type headaches are more than ordinary headaches. They are controlled by the pea-sized pituitary gland, which is one of GOD'S miracles. For whatever reason, these glands decipher, that certain foods and drinks are harmful to you and alerts you to that fact, by shutting down your blood supply. The headaches are caused by the restriction of the tiny capillaries that furnish blood to your brain, located just above the eye. We don't need to know all the intricacies of why and how. All we need to know, is that they will not respond to any pills. The pituitary gland demands that you do not injest these again. You can NOT fool this high level "genius" part of everyone's body. Any amount, no matter how small, such as a particle of chocolate if you allergic to it, will be identified and cause a headache. (I know because I am allergic to chocolate and recently went to bed for three days, because of accidentally eating about a third of a chocolate chip.) Cheese as an example: only one ounce of rennet per thousand pounds of milk is used to color milk to make cheddar cheese. One hundred fifty pounds of cheese is produced from that 1000 pounds and cheddar cheese is a prime headache producer. So the simple answer is; you must identify what your gland doesn't like, and NEVER eat or drink it again.

So the simple answer is; you must identify what YOUR GLAND DOESN'T LIKE, and NEVER eat it again.

And now, I will list all the possible foods and drinks that you MIGHT be affected by. To begin with, there are eight allergens defined by The FDA considered the most common: peanuts, tree nuts, soy, fish, seafood, wheat, eggs, and milk or dairy, as well as any foods that contain gluten. These allergens can cause all kinds of illnesses and some are even fatal, but I am not aware of how any of these cause headaches. I can only speak for myself in that I avoid all nuts and soy products. These are the allergens listed on most food labels. It has recently become mandatory for manufacturers to list MSG in the list of ingredients wherever it is used. You note that food coloring is not among them. The products that affected me the most were:

1.   Food coloring which includes practically all wines, beer, liquors, sodas (except ginger ale and tonic water). It is impossible to list all the foods that contain food coloring. Look for Blue 1 and Blue 6, Red 40 is very common, Green, Yellow 5 and Yellow 6. You may have to rely in looking at the product because of the 2% exemption. FDA exempts manufacturers from identifying any products which constitute less than 2% of the total volume. It is rare that any

coloring would be greater than 2%. You will need to eat only <u>white cheese</u>, as cheddar is colored.

2.   Chocolate in any form.

3.   MSG was a killer for me. Used in all Chinese food products.

4.   Spices except salt, pepper, and cinnamon.

5.   All sugar substitutes such as aspartame. (One of the worst).

6.   Preservatives. Vinegar is probably the basic product that has caused preservatives to be on this list.

7.   Teramines which are produced in manufacturing product includes sausages, wieners and chopped meats.

This is a long list and restricts the diet considerably. However, most people are not allergic to all those mentioned. Most people find they have only one allergen to worry about, probably food coloring being the most prevalent. As most people also know, the peanut allergy is the most deadly and is often fatal.

SUMMARY:

◆ There is no magic pill. Most headaches are not curable, but can be prevented.

◆ Most headaches are preventable, but you must apply the knowledge to isolate the cause.

◆ Take charge of your life. Do not depend on medical advice to do it for you.

◆ You must change your diet to prevent headaches. It demands will power and determination to prevent headaches.

◆ Every headache has a cause and you alone can find it. You must "sweat the little things" for they are most important.

◆ No one can live a normal life with severe headaches, but you can easily live with the preventatives.

◆ FDA-Approved is a misleading term. Means little or nothing to allergy sufferers.

◆ Reading lists of ingredients is a difficult job. Often does not contain info you need.

◆ Liquor and alcohol based products, MSG, sugar substitutes, preservatives, tobacco, chocolate, certain nuts, food coloring, are the principal causes of severe headaches.